MW00990728

Dark Blonde

DARK BLONDE

POEMS ▲ BELLE WARING

Sarabande Books

LOUISVILLE, KENTUCKY

SECOND PRINTING

Managing Editor
Sarabande Books, Inc.
2234 Dundee Road, Suite 200
Louisville, KY 40205

LIBRARY OF CONGRESS CATALOGING-IN-PUBLICATION DATA

Waring, Belle.
    Dark blonde : poems / by Belle Waring. — 2nd. ed.
        p. cm.
    ISBN 1-889330-07-8 (cloth : alk. paper). — ISBN 1-889330-08-6
    (pbk. : alk. paper)
    I. Title.
    PS3573.A7615D37   1997
    811' .54—dc21   96-53105 CIP

Cover painting: Balthus (Balthasar Klossowski de Rola), French, b. 1908, *Solitaire,* oil on canvas, 1943, 161 x 163.9 cm, Joseph Winterbotham Collection, 1964.177 © 1997 Artists Rights Society (ARS), New York/ADAGP, Paris. Photograph © 1996 The Art Institute of Chicago. All rights reserved. Used by kind permission.

Cover and text design by Charles Casey Martin.

Manufactured in the United States of America.
This book is printed on acid-free paper.

Sarabande Books is a nonprofit literary organization.

for my mothers and fathers

Acknowledgments

▲

I am grateful to the editors of the following journals and anthologies for permission to reprint the poems first published therein, sometimes in different versions:

The American Poetry Review: "Use the Following Construction in a Sentence."

The American Voice: "It Was My First Nursing Job," "People Think All Wrong about Manhood."

Between the Heartbeats: Poetry and Prose by Nurses, edited by Cortney Davis and Judy Schaefer, University of Iowa Press: "From the Diary of a Clinic Nurse, Poland, 1945."

Cape Discovery: The Provincetown Fine Arts Work Center Anthology, edited by Bruce Smith and Catherine Gammon, Sheep Meadow Press: "Twenty-Four-Week Preemie, Change of Shift."

Cimarron Review: "He Said Yes," "So Get over It, Honey."

For a Living: The Poetry of Work, edited by Nicholas Coles and Peter Oresick, University of Illinois Press: "Before Penicillin."

Green Mountains Review: "From the Diary of a Prisoner's Nurse, Mississippi, 1972," "The Brothers on the Trash Truck and My Near-Death Experience."

Hayden's Ferry Review: "Look," "On First Hearing T'ao Ch'ien," "Pick It Up."

Indiana Review: "Ending Green," "Fever, Mood, and Crows," "So What Would You Have Done?"

Nebraska Review: "Baltazar Beats His Tutor at Scrabble," "Eleventh Day of Rain."

Saltimbanquers: "To Them, to Their First Conversation."

The Southern Review: "In the Ladies' Room at the Honeybee Bar and Grille," "Late in the Teachers' Lounge."

Things Shaped in Passing: More "Poets for Life" Writing from the AIDS Pandemic, edited by Michael Klein and Richard McCann, Persea Books: "For My Third Cousin Ray John."

TriQuarterly: "An Engine Fire over the Ocean Compared to the Suburbs," "The Forgery," "Jasmine Dreams," "You Could Have Been Me."

I would like to thank the National Endowment for the Arts, the D.C. Commission on the Arts and Humanities, and the Virginia Center for the Creative Arts for fellowships that helped me complete these poems.

Thanks to Sarah Gorham, Jeffrey Skinner, and the staff at Sarabande.

Je vous remercie profondement: Lisa Bahlinger, Michael Burkard, Frank Dunn, Rachel Eisler, Jose Funes, Catherine Gammon, Emmy and Arnold Jacobius, Mona Kanin, Judith Podell, Denise Schooling, Michael Trombley, Chris Wallin, Kent Waring, Bruce Weigl, Tony Whedon, David Wojahn, and Franz Wright.

Contents

▲

I cannot tell if the day
is ending, or the world, or if
the secret of secrets is inside me again.
        —Anna Akhmatova

Another is searching in the mud for bones, rinds.
How to write, after that, about the infinite?
        —César Vallejo

Dark Blonde

SURE I DO

I've already drowned—so, green-song of eyes,
how could the flames in your river make me
turn

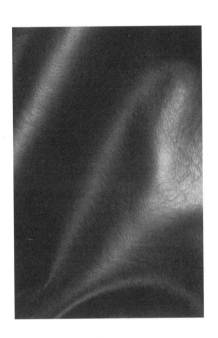

LOOK

Your street at sundown.
Your window, the only one lit up

in all those apartments
stacked silhouette black

against the sky—what a color!
like Sargasso—

loud, like they threw blue dye in it.
Citizen, look up,

the sky god is speaking.
Man, that blue is talking:

You on the old old earth,
listen to me, don't blast yourself.

There: the woman on your balcony.
The woman you let slip—

her forearms on the railing
letting the breeze mess with her sleeves.

Behind her in the room
the books unbend

hover off the shelves
and like a small space station

they wheel like electrons in her skirt—
the books open up to the lines you want

open like air
like water that opens wherever you already are.

Man, look up. Even a small child
has sense enough to drink that blue

whose beauty wounds him so precisely
he knows his life is worth saving.

and I was stupid in it. I thought a doctor would not be unkind.
One wouldn't wait for a laboring woman to dilate to ten cm.

He'd brace one hand up his patient's vagina,
clamp the other on her pregnant belly, and force the fetus

through an eight-centimeter cervix.
She tore, of course. Bled.

Stellate lacerations extend from the cervix
like an asterisk. The staff nurses stormed and hissed

but the head nurse shrugged, *He doesn't like to wait around.*
No other doctor witnessed what he did. The man was an elder

in his church. He chattered and smiled broadly as he worked.
He wore the biggest gloves we could stock.

It was my first real job and I was scared in it.
One night a patient of his was admitted

bleeding. The charge nurse said, *He won't rip her.*
You take this one.

So I took her.
She quickly delivered a dead baby boy.

Not long dead—you could tell by the skin, intact.
But long enough.

When I wrapped him in a blanket, the doctor flipped open the cover
to let the mother view the body, according to custom.

The baby lay beside her.
He lay stretched out and still.

What a pity, the doctor said.
He seized the baby's penis between his own forefinger and thumb.

It was the first time I had ever seen a male not circumcised
and I was taken aback by the beauty of it.

Look, said the doctor, *A little boy. Just what we wanted.*
His hand, huge on the child, held the penis as if he'd found

a lovecharm hidden in his grandmother's linen.
And then he dropped it.

The mother didn't make a sound.
When the doctor left, she said to me in a far flat voice

I called and told him I was bleeding bad.
He told me not to worry.

I don't remember what I said. Just that
when I escorted her husband from the lobby

the doctor had already gone home. The new father followed me
with a joyful strut. I thought *Sweet Jesus Christ*

—*Did the doctor speak to you?*
—*No ma'am,* the father said.

I said quick-as-I-could-so-I-wouldn't-have-to-think—
The baby didn't make it.

The man doubled over. I told him all wrong.
I would do it all over again.

Say—
Please, sir. Sit down. I'm so very sorry to tell you—

No. It's been sixteen years.
I would say, *I am your witness.*

No. I have never told the whole truth.
Forgive me.

It was my first job
and I was lost in it.

AN ENGINE FIRE OVER THE OCEAN COMPARED TO THE SUBURBS

You wake up and the world looks strange...
—Fernando Pessoa

I was calm the day after—trying to tell Jasmine how the engine burned at 25,000 feet, over the North Atlantic and dark, how the big jet lurched as the pilot dumped his fuel and outside my window, the twelve tongues of Lucifer—fire.

And next to me, a baby boy on his father's lap so I held the child's gaze and he made no cry. He wasn't fooling. Now how can I thank him, dark the baby's eyes holding me up—

Jasmine says, STOP! It's just that post-traumatic stress—just relax, we'll rent a movie.

And I'm trying to tell her, calmly: How can you rent a movie with this *light* everywhere.

Jasmine says, *Light?*

Light isn't *around* things—it *is* things.

Jasmine's a nurse with three small kids and no metaphysical leanings, and in her backyard lives an orphan desert tortoise some forest ranger gave her. I carried out a bowl of raw green beans and sat in the serene suburban grass.

The tortoise ambled over. He opened his primeval beak—exposing a horrible wet pink tongue—then accepted snap beans with stately gusto.

I was trying to tell Jasmine, you wake up and the world looks exquisitely strange—

But what's an engine fire compared to the suburbs?

Tortoises live a hundred years, probably because they don't take plane rides. I patted this one on his variegated shell, that fabulous bulk that felt both foreign and very close—like something from a planet too far away to see, like something of myself—and we stayed like that in the signifying grass and watched it blaze around us like the sea.

IN THE LADIES' ROOM AT THE HONEYBEE BAR AND GRILLE

Jean sticks that stuff in her arm again.
Makes her eyes glint like a scot-free fox. But man—
she's not.

Tipples on Lodonia's flask
and Lodonia's murderous.
Her uncle raped her sister, right, so Lodonia's copped a .22
snugged in her black clutch bag.
Brushes the hair back out of my eyes.

Jean Ann! she says, *Touch this child with a needle*
and I'll kick your lame white ass!

I watch her strut. The color of Lodonia—
color of high tide sand. She got kitkat eyes.
One time she got thrown down the Honeybee's back steps,
bit clean through her lip and never cried.

Now the band's crazing up
into jazz so frax and dissonant the audience bellows. They want
love songs. As for us, we're safe in the Ladies'
but my eyes in the glass—too scared to leave the Ladies' room,
first time ever on the street, scared to smell Lodonia's flask,
tugging that liquory reek

like my dad, I'd spot him sharp across the room—
his face stuck to the mask booze makes.

Now the band lurches into "My Favorite Things"
when the door slaps open and a queen trips in on fat platform heels
and a turquoise shift above the knee.

He says, *Hey honey.* I say, *Hey* back.
But Lodonia balks. Man doesn't see, he just scrapes off
his two-tone wig, rubs water all over his scalp.
Inside his arms all bumps and sores track up and down.
The color of him—stale strong coffee down your dress.
Six shades darker than Lodonia.

This the Ladies' room, she says, *You nigger faggot—*

Then the man stands up.
Water ribbles down his face and his eyes snatch at you like a baby
trying to tell you what happened.

It was just one word
one single word

Cunt, he said.

When the gun came out he said, *Please*

Please

I wish I could say
that I kept both my hands on Lodonia's arm
say nobody got hurt
I wish I could say
come up a bad cloud
and washed down the walls of my face

Say I wish I could say
I am not the only one who never did time
and did survive
and I remember much better than my own

that man's eyes

SO GET OVER IT, HONEY

First bout of Shanghai flu, sweat the bed without you
First night walking west over Ellington Bridge
spy Marilyn's face in the mural over HEIDI'S LIQUOR,
yearning, so I say, *Don't kill yourself* but this is ridiculous
without you
First conversation with my mother who tells me I'm selfish
without you
First movie I see, matinee about Monk whose wife and mistress
looked after him so he could play but still he cracked, he was a
genius without you
First Dorito binge 'til my lips turn into the slugs I poured salt on
when I was a kid without you
First talk-the-talk with Dave who says you're a schmuck so I
should go get laid without you
First drive to Carolina where my cousin Mason's wife takes the babies
and leaves the state and he crawls into detox—not easy, but simple
without you
First Christmas I wish I was Buddhist without you
First death, it was Dom, he was twenty-seven, lung cancer and that's
    all I know
without you
First time I tutor the kids at the shelter and say, *Tell me what you
    like to do*
and one says, *Go see Grandma* & the other says, *Stupid! Grandma's
    dead*
without you
First January thaw, I find a 1943 penny in the alley without you

First period, Oh there is a God without you

USE THE FOLLOWING
CONSTRUCTION IN A SENTENCE

Tu
me
manques

No
Nobody misses you—Me
I'm like the French the wary French

They say instead of "I miss you"
Tu me manques
You me lack

You're like the time
I stood at the blackboard 'til I cried and finally the teacher smirks
You can never divide by zero, she says, *Trick question—sit down*

Tu me manques
You are lacking
to me

I'm like the French
cool thinky French
There are some things I best not say

But it's safe to recount
how balletically you rode a ten-speed
the one abandoned on the street

and how you proposed before even one kiss
and how, September, when your visa came through
that red lipsticky stamp cost you

15

It cost
    So you bolt
    I break down

Then one evening, months later, this other fellow
takes me to hear a string ensemble playing Bach
like a beast with its multicolored arms rippling the rarefied light

and it makes me cry
so my hot new herringbone date pipes up
You're such a sensitive girl

Tu me manques
You
lack me

I went to a reception
It was a mistake
The councilman tried to corner me by the artist's print of the
    Kurdish dead

and there was no *you*
to shoot a look to
telegraph for help

so I said, *Roll call! Excusez-moi!*
Dumped my cranberry punch on his ego-shined shoes
You shoulda seen me cuttin' that move

You
lack
me

Once I got home I hunkered down in my swarthy kitchen
and read some poems my student sent
and I know as I talk out of my own bones

she'll be a hit
and I'll live to see it
She lacks me not

Such a lot of things around here you'd like to glimpse
My cousin Karnay got a brand new beau
He sings right up from the roots of his feet

that kiss-me-all-over-'til-the-birds-crank-up kinda scat
You'd hit it off
You could jam all night

but you wouldn't want to come back
I'd cut clean around you like a bad accident
that the state trooper waves me right past

You lack
man
you lack

Things happen round here
that you would cry at the beauty of
you would shout

like I'm in the Metro waiting to change
I see an Amish family get on the train
and as the young girl turns

and spies me through the glass
there on her face the most searing joy
so I wave to her

and she
without hesitating
waves back

You lack me
You're like trying to divide by zero
after everybody says

You can't
I'm like the French
the luscious French

playing those cornball accordions in the street
so they don't have to say
Come back

THE BROTHERS ON THE TRASH TRUCK AND MY NEAR-DEATH EXPERIENCE

Having just been left for good by you—your tongue
flicking over your lips like a thirsty newt, your cheeks plush with
    screwery—
having been left so, I walked into the backing-up path of a trash truck.

Its ding-reverse bell must have been defunct.
It was the side-rider's *YO!* that halted it.
Don't hurt her baby, don't hurt her! the side-rider called in a
    franticky chant.

The driver leapt out.
MISS, MISS! cried the side-rider, *MISS!*
You were nowhere in sight. There I lay in my neighbor's hedge,

outlandishly unhurt. I looked up. The driver had
green eyes, a tall tan black man with those farfetched
feline eyes, like say maybe

one of his foremothers volunteered for a shot at the Nordic gene pool,
or, on the other hand, consider that one etymology of *motherfucker*
cites masters raping female slaves, the children forced to watch...

but is this my business how the man got green eyes?
I'm glad I had this thought because I don't know what to do with it.
Forgive me, I said. *My boyfriend dumped me, I wasn't looking...*

We were shook—me, driver, side-rider
by the divine simplicity of the Near Miss.
So they took me home. The brothers escorted me back—

two blocks cruising high in the cab
like the Empress of Metropolis.
Don't even worry 'bout it, the driver said,

If he don't come back, go on and catch you a bigger fish.
And the side-rider meanwhile
leapt and landed and kept on leaping,

on and off the rolling truck, heaving those garbage bins
light as confetti, light as burned billets-doux,
the sweet spent tickets to my heart.

BEFORE PENICILLIN

to the memory of E. S. Waring, M.D.

The doctor steps into the shack.

> Light
> is December dusk. Sleet clouds
> bunched up.

All the beds are here in this one room
pushed up against the wall
and even from across the room and even in the shambling light
her face—

> Mask-like. Greenish-gray.
> The facies of impending death.

The parents
pull up a straight-backed chair for him.

He takes the hand of a child he delivered
fourteen years ago.

> Her pulse is a thread
> so thin it would fray if you blew on it.

It's all right, Evie.

Then he folds the army blanket down.

> The girl's entire abdomen is abscessed.
> Burst appendix rotting for days and now spread.

He listens to her chest,
tucks the blanket back under her chin.

She opens her mouth and the
smell

It is 1933.
There is no such thing as penicillin.

Let me get her to the hospital—

No Sir, the father says. *You take her over there, she'll die.*

They quarrel until the mother says PLEASE
once, then is still.

       When the doctor finally steps outside,
       he can hear the younger children begin to keen.

He tugs the brim of his hat down low.
His wife will be angry again, at him and the house
and the bank in town which has filed to foreclose
and their four small girls whiny with colds and the sleet
which will needle him wicked *thwik*
on the road and in the ditch the nine miles home.

       He can hear the younger children begin to scream.

He washes his hands on the bristling grass,
runs them under his mare's black mane and
leans on her neck—

       on her fragrant, inculpable neck.

▲

FROM THE DIARY OF A CLINIC
NURSE, POLAND, 1945

> *The only safe conclusion to be drawn from the multitude of*
> *reports is that life in dark closets, wolves' dens, forests or*
> *sadistic parents' backyards is not conducive to good health*
> *and normal development.*
> —from "Wolf Children" in *The Genesis of Language*,
> edited by Frank Smith and George A. Miller

Alone with the child, I lay down to bare my neck like a dog
surrendering.

The linguists will use her to theorize on the origins of speech—of
which she now has none. I'd like to bathe her without being flayed by
those six-year-old teeth.

Female child found abandoned in thick woods, healthy, but feral, feet
indurated. Hearing intact.

Bays like a wolf.

When I speak, her eyes turn curious. Even dogs grasp simple commands,
and she is, *a priori,* more intelligent than they. *Marie,* I call her, after
Curie, who took two Nobels, chemistry and physics.

The doctors note Semitic traits: deep-hooded eyes, a certain nose,
hair dark whorls reduced now to a bramble mat half down her back.
To save her from the camps, someone must have led her deep into the
woods to wander there like Gretel. Like Snow White.

Doctor Krynski tells his students how Rome's founders were two
brothers suckled by a wolf. But this girl isn't founding Rome. Red
Army men brought her in this week, naked under the sergeant's coat.
At least they hadn't raped—still, her howls raised the hair on my neck.

Marie, I say, and she *looks* at me, as if the syllables *meant* something.

Start with the resonant consonant, *M*—lips meet, then release. *Muh. Marie.*

Dirty Jew, the night nurse says, right to her face. The child knows the tone, growls back and bites until they order chloral hydrate. When she wakes up scrubbed and shorn like Sampson, her eyes say, *Thou hast betrayed me.*

My studies in physics have been blasted of course, and now the doctors snap at me as if I were their serf tending pigs.

But I am not a simple nurse.

Alone with the child, I lay down to bare my neck like a dog surrendering and for the first time she crouched near enough to sniff me. Then the neurologist barged in, and, finding us on the floor like that, had a jealous snit. The grunting little academic—he wants her for research, but first he must examine her—and this she won't permit. He'd have to drug her—and drugged, she won't react.

I gave her an orange whirligig, I swear I heard her laugh: a hoarse, exotic yelp.

Muh, I said. *Marie.*

I lay on the floor like a pup at play. I lay there and begged the Blessed Virgin for Her help and was seized quite suddenly with weeping. The child fixed me with a concentrated stare, then crawled over and sniffed my hand: carbolic soap and tears, if indeed these have a scent.

More doctors came and she fled then to her corner as they shouted at my lack of dignity.

I need the work. I did not shout back.

Marie, you see me, how I'll soon turn twenty-three and have no sweetheart, family dead, mind matted up and useless and scared for you, Marie of the woods so thick no one heard you shriek. I have not seen your parental wolves but I've heard them howling at the lone, callipygous moon, wolves trapped down here in this wrong life. Wrong continent. Wrong earth.

▲

BALTAZAR BEATS HIS TUTOR AT
SCRABBLE

If Myra counts fifteen cows and Alfredo counts nine,
how many more cows did Myra count?

Baltazar counts on his fingers.
I wish I could stay here 'til morning, he says—cool,

matter-of-fact. Thirteen, sixth grade. All this week
he's been late. Lip swollen and split. *I have nightmares,* he says,

Like falling. Pours out a Scrabble shower of blonde wood Chiclets.
Crow-black hair, square competent hands. Two grades behind.

Ten points for a Z, Baltazar. I spell PASS.
He spells ZAP on the Triple Word Score, has to multiply by three.

—*You tell your mom you can't sleep?*
—*She lets me lie on the sofa and watch TV.*

I spell ZOUNDS—God's wounds, a Shakespearean oath:
Zounds, I was never so bethumpt with words.

Baltazar doesn't forget where he's from, how beautiful it is
and how fraught. In a flurry of Spanish he spells

MUCHACHO then GRITO then spells I GET UP AT FIVE TO
    HAUL THE WASH
DOWN TO 14TH AND V, HAVE IT HOME FOLDED BEFORE
    DAD WAKES UP

'CAUSE MOM IS ALREADY GONE TO WORK.
I spell DID HE BUST YOUR LIP

The odder the letter, the higher the score.
He spells I WANT TO STAY HERE 'TIL NIGHT PUTS ITS
   HANDS IN THE AIR

Blanks spell what you like—you rub them like luck,
the polished wood suave as a horse's neck.

Blanks goof around—propped in your eye sockets, you squint
like smiling against the sun on the skirts of the mountains,

on your grandmother's face, calm, waking you up.
On the words she would sing, and the music not separate from them.

PEOPLE THINK ALL WRONG ABOUT MANHOOD

When I met Jacob, he'd just escaped a police state.
Scrawny white guy, he talked all jacked up on nicotine,
laughed like a .22
crak-crak echo in the alley. Eyes
you already know about—how they undercut

this dodobird reception chat, where Jacob looks forty-five, except
at me—eyes like a kid who gets hit.
Hit. Then they tell him
Strip. And nobody calls the cops.
Because they are the cops.

I got a cat with six toes per foot who can smell the landlord
down the block. Jacob thinks I'm a sentimentalist.

So what. This past winter I worked just enough to pay my rent,
lived on greens and greasy cornbread, slept with the light and the radio on
so no one would think I was alone. I had bad dreams where I found
little boys in a cold steel sink, face down on a wire brush.
A dusky pulse threads one boy's arm. They have been
sexually tortured
then shadows grease over the windows and
the door   *no lock*

I would wake up seized with a sick headache,
and lose whole days like that.

Jacob says there's no such thing as love at first sight.
You all know the lightning bolt—

Juliet and Romeo. But this is no
play. One morning after I hadn't slept

a silver stretch limo
nearly hit me in the alley where the neighbor kids hang
and the pigeons peck over the cobblestones,
when here comes this limo
with its minky black windows all rolled up tight so you can't name
     names
and the sucker never even slowed down. Made me jump back,
skin my hand on the door of the shed.

I wanted to live
after that.

There's a park near my place
where the creek cuts the city clean down to the river.
Sunlight mottles the poplars, aggie-eyes the small water.
If you toss cat chow to those citified ducks, you draw
mamas in camouflage, splendid green heads,
a white rascal like Donald minus jacket and cap,
shimmying his dignified tush.

Ducks are appointed by God to give doofy people a safe date.

We walked through the city
counting up different riffs that we heard on the street—
boom boxes, radios, churches, jukes
girls jumping double Dutch
boys drumming drywall buckets in their sidewalk *batería*
a twelve-piece band of trombones and a tuba
a guy slamming cups of spare change for percussion
—count 'em up.

Get twelve tunes, go on home

and there the man next door plays Villa-Lobos on piano
'til he hits a change and splatters jazz riffs that feel like the rush
you get in a plane when the glaze-blue day pops out of the murk

then you're back inside and Jacob is just somewhere
quiet in the house with you.

These moments are underrated because they're not a Pepsi commercial
—no big male teeth, no young women with important hair.

Things quite silently
shift.

And when a man is brave enough
to cry whatever he's saved up—
you recognize him.

And you—you save up what comes
after he's finished his crying.

HE SAID YES

Some days I crave my graceful beau
I used to talk to by the ocean
where the light was the beam-o hyaline light
even the blind when they die shall see.

He insisted on things—he wasn't shy.
I said, No. I wasn't ready.
He said, Yes. And I let him, but still
I was scared. A lot of people have this problem.

Granted, some words look right sharp on the page,
sure of themselves as assassins, but to read out loud
as sad as you feel in a voice all clotted up I think is
brave. I hope I am that brave. Now

some things I have learned to do: I will never
kill myself. There are ways
to grieve that do work.
So now. Sun's out.

And here you come, girl, strolling down Seventh Street
grinning like a choo-choo, like you're all of eleven,
your old man's teaching you to box step, and before he leans in
and porks his tongue into your mouth—

before that—
there's a moment
you are actually
happy.

BIPOLAR AFFECTIVE DISORDER AS POSSIBLE ADAPTIVE ADVANTAGE

You should have seen those mountains, cousin.
Tidal waves of frozen rock like huge implacable parents.

I buried a poem at the base of a tree. I wanted nothing—
no food no drink—just to write one thing on top of another.
I just wanted not to be scared of old Mr. Madness skulldugging around
sporting his diamond stubble
and on my way home, there he was—
standing in the train between two cars
on the floor plates shifting in a racket ever faster
as the train blasted into another country altogether.

I see it, cousin.
You and I had a common ancestor, time out of mind,
somebody with a mad talent for the trance,
for collapsing onto the rusty ground, for tasting the old
blood of the earth.

If you fell down raving, the tribe would attend you—
you'd wake with song-stories to make pictures in the mind.

Without those gifts, the manic-depressed
would have been just a fractious pain in the ass
and get pitched off a cliff.

The tribe would survive and they'd get to keep the art—
a thousand notes to call the ancestors back to the root.

At the onset of mania, Robert Lowell told his wife,
I can feel it in the spine. It's a funny creeping feeling . . .
coming up the spine from the lower back up.

Cousin, there's no romance in this.
So this is it. We're obliged now to survive
whether or not we still hear the green music we heard as babies
when Nanny held us fast so we'd calm down
and watch the window change to night.

The night was birds changing to wind.
The night all along was feeding us.

The night was a hum and a pulse in her chest
and the hurt escaping her marrow bones
from the hollow the madness had left.

LATE IN THE TEACHERS' LOUNGE

So I ask,
How many of you know someone who's been shot?
And half the class puts their hands up.

O April, bless them—
O bless me, tulips, you cuds of color,
I'd like to swallow you whole.

And I'm just goofy enough to do that—
you should see my remedial class sit up.
But!

Those tulips he gave me, those purplish clots—now *there's*
a right foxy stunt.
Thank God he doesn't *look* heroic.

Be*cause,* girlfriend, a crush is no reason to lose one's insolence!
As a man he belongs to the scurrilous tribe
that cheated my unhappy mother.

O tulips, bless me.
His lips are the pillows a pilgrim sinks into and finds
God on the spot.

God, don't let him get shot!
'Cause phalanxes of tulips are kicking the can-can
out in the woozy dark.

34

TWENTY-FOUR-WEEK PREEMIE, CHANGE OF SHIFT

We're running out of O$_2$
screaming down the Southwest Freeway in the rain
the nurse-practitioner and me
rocking around in the back of an ambulance
trying to ventilate a preemie with junk for lungs
when we hit
rush hour

     Get us the hell out of here

You bet the driver said
and pulled right onto the median strip
with that maniacal glee they get

I was too scared for the kid and drunk with the speed
—the danger didn't feel like danger at all
it felt like love—to worry about *my* life
Fuck that

     Get us back to Children's so we can put a chest tube in
        this kid

And when we got to the unit
the attending physician—Loretta—was there
and the nurses
the residents
they save us

Loretta plants her stethoscope on the kid's chest
and here comes the tech driving the portable

like it's a Porsche
Ah Jesus he says

The baby's so puny he could fit on your dinner plate

X-ray says the tech
and everybody backs up
except for Loretta
so the tech drapes a lead shield over her chest

X-RAY! says the tech

There's a moment after he cones down the lens
just before he shoots

You hold your breath
You forget
what's waiting
back at your house

Nobody blinks
poised for that sound
that radiological *meep*

and Loretta with her scrub top on backwards
so you can't peep down to her peanutty boobs
Loretta with her half-Chinese, half-Trinidadian
half-smile

Loretta, all right, ambu-bagging the kid
never misses a beat
calm and sharp as a mama-cat who's just kicked the dog's butt
now softjaws her kitten out of the ditch

There's a moment
you can't even hear the bag

puffing
quick quick quick

Before the tech shoots
for just that second
I quit being scared
I forget to be scared

God

How can people abandon each other?

▲

FROM THE DIARY OF A PRISONER'S NURSE, MISSISSIPPI, 1972

We had her open into the uterus
down to the bag of waters still intact around the baby—
floating, oblivious, asleep.
Oh! the surgeon said. I had never
heard one of his kind sound so innocent, surprised. Never seen
the womb laid open to a fetus sleeping head-up in its home—

translucent sac. But you can't stand around all night
like Biblical shepherds, dumb with adoration. The surgeon has to
shred the bag—glistening surgical birth. Now

go back
to the bag of waters and its cloudy light, silvery mizzle
like March rain at midday and the light way back behind it.

Light in prison can be like that, skim, before sunup,
gray to bluish where they found her in labor, tetanic contractions,
the uterine muscle stretched morbidly thin, the baby

breech, head palpable as a cat under an old quilt, something
wrong, her first baby, the woman screaming and the inmates, louder,
screaming over her *Get a doctor!*

Uterine rupture. A basket splitting from the weight of its fruit.
She was twenty-one. Wheat. Wax. Dust. How
we got the kid out, I don't know—the surgeon was slow as an old cur.

She just bled out.
After, the doctor offered me a smoke
which I took to avoid letting him catch me in the eye.

The eyes of the dying sometimes glaze over like cloudy plastic
stretched over a window to thwart the rain—the film of it
fuzzes the light. The old eyes of the scrub nurse, eyes over the mask,

sad cynic: *Give it up.* They didn't try to save the mother.
One year out of school, I would not obey, went for the anesthesia cart,
albumin in drawer three—

then her pressure—the bottom dropped out.
I couldn't get her back. The baby screamed at birth.
The baby screamed at birth.

▲

THE FORGERY

—For uncrossmatched blood, the doctor must sign.

I said, It's for a baby! Stabbed in utero! *I'll* sign for the doctor.

—You mean *forge* it? Forget it.

The woman behind the blood bank counter then tapped on the page with her index finger, with her salon-painted nail, tuff as an escutcheon—tiny gold griffin on a field of carmine. O she had a haughty eye.

—*Physician's* signature, she said.

—Where's your supervisor?

—I *am* the supervisor. And I'm not losing my job 'cause a *you.*

And since no pity would move her, nor rank, nor threat, and a legal signature meant lost minutes, and since the baby was preemie, the baby was shocky, and it was four in the morning, gall of the night, I saw fit to go crazy.

—*Lose your job? Who'd want it?* I got two babies up there on *vents* already, and now *this* one, *surprise!* The mother walks into the ER, collapses, with multiple stab wounds, belly fulla blood, but when they take her to the OR and open her up *there's this twenty-eight-week fetus inside.* So they STAT-page us and the shit hits—*OK?* But you know why I like it? You get an admission, that crazy first hour, everybody works together, everybody helps you out, and you reach a point—not out of the woods, but you're getting there, *you feel it*— and somebody cracks a joke. You look up—you all laugh. *That* moment. *Help me,* I said.

She turned her back. Walked away. On the wall someone had stuck a poster:

IT HAS COME TO THE ATTENTION OF THE MANAGEMENT THAT EMPLOYEES EXPIRING ON THE JOB ARE FAILING TO FALL DOWN. ANYONE WHO REMAINS DEAD IN AN UPRIGHT POSITION WILL BE DROPPED FROM THE PAYROLL.

Then she was back. Plunked down two pints of blood.

—Sign, she said.

So I signed, I forged, I grabbed the two units, uncrossmatched blood, color of garnets, color of beets, hugged the blood to my chest and I ran all three flights and I ran, never tired, the talker, the forger, I ran with the gorgeous, ran with the anonymous, ran with cold dark blood.

ON FIRST HEARING T'AO CH'IEN

for Tony

I'm a strong girl—been to the desert with a puggish backpack,
waiting for the rain, my nose in a book, waiting for my life
to show up, my eyes like critters ticking over the print,
looking for the magic bullet in the words,
the curing pellet, the trip tab,
the launching pad—
I read too much.
I've been like this
since I was a kid, a midge, a sprout,
learning to read soon as I could talk, pointing
right to the word soon as folks called it out: RABBIT—
picture gave it away: white dude up on his two hind legs,
witty ears, overalls. I'd rather read than eat, but rabbit knows much
    better
than that. Which is why I'm here on a Saturday night, no date, none
    in sight.

So when Whedon calls up
to read me T'ao Ch'ien's "Elegy for Myself,"
it feels like 1971, crossing the Painted Desert
in a old panel truck. I and the others still had hope—Nixon
wasn't yet reelected. The earth was painted hilarious rose, ochery red.
When we stop for gas, stand on the ground beside the Ford, *The
    world is boundless,*
boundless—and above, underbellies of cumulus heaps reflecting
the earth's ruddling pink. Better than acid. Seventeen,
I've escaped my home—my death is behind me.
I am the rabbit who tricks the trap,
abides in the breeze to tell.

FEVER, MOOD, AND CROWS

Crow talks.
His second, down the alley, picks it up.

Crows have a language
which I learned passively the winter I got sick.

Feverish off and on for weeks
then slung in a depressive mesh, gray and translucent as a caul,

I was as close as I had ever been to signing myself in and letting the
     nurses
hook me up.

Everyone real was off at work. The street was lull, I lived alone.
I lay still and half-listened to the crows. Their parlay

was impossible to crack. Then one day I came to and realized
It has layers. Like any language. So first, get the rhythm of it.

Late March. The surly part of winter you want over with, the part
that recurs. Relapses. That keeps fucking you up.

I guess I thought about hurting myself.
This is a mood and time that crows defy.

Late March. Pusillanimous rain on trees shut bare against the wind
on a branch by my window where a crow sits, the crow who's just

woken me up. Woken me not tentatively, not clearing his throat
to check on incoming weather. No, this crow's *furious*—

his kaa-kaa relentless, kaa-kaa machine gun,
his kaa-kaa typed onto the page scans entirely stressed. All

accents—kaa-kaa streams like anarchists. He will not
shut up.

I slap open the window. It's freezing. He spots me.
OK! I say. *I'm up!*

The crow clamps shut his double-hinged beak
and we exchange a measuring stare.

Watching snug from your car on your way to work
you would've seen a woman riddled, half nuts,

shouting out her window at the air. You might have felt a chill and
jacked the heat all the way up.

Nemo censetur ignorare legem.
No one is presumed ignorant of the law. But crow is a law un-

to himself. Anyway, he had reason.
Anyway, he won—

the woman did live. Because the woman
got up.

HEAR ME, OH MY GRANDMOTHERS

With a blind date
I went to the prom in ecru satin and an ice-blue sash
cut from my grandmother's breath.

Six gowns she wore, one on top of another
fleeing the Czar
to Sebastopol
Cuba
the Bronx
where she worked her way up to Inspector of Lace
and was then blacklisted as a socialist.
The sweatshop
turns the eyes to lightning spokes.

The war hit, she worked in hospitals, she worked like mules
so I wouldn't have to (queued up, as I was, to be born)

but see now, Nana, your girl's gone soft—
if she misses a meal her knees start to knock,
the only thing she's good for is talk talk talk. Even at the prom
she was too shy to dance up a frank sweat.

Sweatshop light—it throttles the eyes.

From where you are, Nana, among the dead,
do you see my life, squanderous and forked,
middle-aged, plump, flinging birdseed in the garden
as a storm bulls up?

A soldier of the Czar received a monthly ration
—sunflower seeds which fed man and bird alike
could be scattered on the graves that the dead might rest.

Now my bones say this:

Nana, who is like you?

This lightning—
it was cut from my grandmother's breath.

JASMINE DREAMS

My sleep is the color of burnt grapes
I dream I'm awake
I dream the phone rings I pick it up

Must be Jasmine got thrown out by her husband
Stay here, girleen, we'll get dressed up
Bring your paloozy dresses, your red brassiere
Paint palm trees on my fingernails

But no it's not Jasmine it's my father in the dream
calling in the dropwell of night
slurry and pissed

He wants something, what is it

Then he's in the room with me
handing over my sister's baby
who regards me with an eye of shimmering slate
opens his mouth with no teeth and says

You're holding me all wrong, OK?

But Jasmine has worthier dreams

She sees the politically murdered
and the disappeared
the mutilated

Her nightmares make mine look suburban
since mine are only the weirdness of my father's voice
which I cannot explain in the middle of the night

when Jasmine finally calls
for real now

because they're walking the halls again
halls the color of burnt coffee

SHOTS

Three nurses to hold him, this four-year-old who kicks me
crazy in the belly—six months pregnant but *ha!*
I've got the needle—the Measles-Mumps-Rubella.
Child, it stings like hell.

Listen to me, my little immunized enemy—
I'll take a bruise from you
before I'll see another kid like the one carried through the clinic doors
at the end of shift in his father's arms, seizing
seizing
The father's shirt is
black with sweat
is praying in Mexican

grand mal, I try to get a line in, Mother of God, intractable
Get him over to St. Luke's

but in the ambulance, he codes, and then, in the ER
with the furious swirl of personnel, crash cart rumbling up, curtains
snatched to shield him from the drive-bys and the drunks,
the boy expired.
Measles encephalitis.
He never got his shots.

So walk out, dark blonde, into the sun that will scald you red
and bleach your hair to tungsten burning, drive the dusty valley
    smacked with
irrigated fields. Bad counterfeit. Too green.

His young bones green, unripe, *gronjo*
from the old Teutonic root—

Green. Untrained. Green. Freshly killed.
His young bones green and full of marrow.

Green at work there in the rows, hands stretched out to pick a
beefsteak tomato at the end of season when they strip the plants clean
whether the fruit is ripe or not.

WAITING TO BE TOLD I'M NO GOOD

Here is the dirt space
And you have always known about this

It's the gap in conversation
—the shift

A man will cough
a woman look away

at what's coming to the point
the intricate snatch to the solar plexus

May we speak to you
you dead cube whirling

and the one grain on the side of the scale
that clatters on stone scrapes burns bloody

homunculus
eyes raked to slits

my unculus
full weight

it wouldn't stop
it woke me up

PARTS

I went to see Woodson
knucklebone dice knocking inside my head

I went to find him
my first
my flood
and me rolling into dice down that hospital hall
skidding right into the *she*
not me
not grated and spaced
not visiting my first

Woodson
in seclusion
four-corner restraints
strapped to his Veterans' Hospital bed
smelling of undigested blood

He was calm by then

Me the one with eyes like houseflies beating their heads on the glass

Four days on his back in cowhide restraints
The nurse refused to unstrap him

I went to the Ladies'
let my head down sick
and a woman with red hair longer than her skirt
came into the stall and wiped my face

It's your man?

He's broke down, I said

And me turning nineteen
Woodson my first
taught me to work on his Chevy truck
pull plug wires and watch for sparks
jack it up, break the lugs
so I wouldn't get stranded and have some redneck
knock me in the head or crush my fingers
crack my piano hands

Take your time now, he said
Saw a man lose his fingers 'cause he wouldn't wait

So wait, he told me that when he was fourteen—
I didn't know him then, I couldn't save him then—
on a flat back road on a wet June night
this cracker whipped out two feet of pipe
and porked him in the ass

There was no one to tell

So tell

So four years later
he gets shipped out

Vietnam
right before Tet

Infantry means right out of high school
he gets to hold his buddy whose legs are blown off to the groin

He gets to panic
shoot before he looks

He hit a little girl

And the dice in my head say
You're just a black and white leaflet
that didn't stop the war

Woodson
in seclusion

Let him up, I said

He had eyes like Tobias when he meets the Angel
eyes the slur molassey ache
steam and wait
Woodson listened, never held his breath impatient
for his own turn to speak

Listen

My father, he'd shoved his fist inside a voice
in a train jumping the track down my gullet

So, so listen
he heard me
my first
Woodson
my shout
my tight wood grain on the roof of the piano's mouth

He tore the door off its hospital hinges
and got shipped downstate

And when today rattles back down in my head
it seems I'm forty
and this guy from the want ad's here to sell me his truck
so I tie on a headrag, slide underneath
and see his secret oil leaks talking to the street

He says, *Look at the pretty lady jumping under my truck*

54

I crawled out with the flashlight in my fist

Get this waste off my block

And my inside eye spied Woodson
smiling over some resuscitated engine
and the dice rolled up real tight in my head—

You know he broke down
'cause you just didn't love him enough

And I saw his eyes
and my breath
snapped
like the green bone
in a child's arm

like the fist that hits you with what you have finally lost

SO WHAT WOULD YOU HAVE DONE?

On the train to D.C., a priest sat beside me, and outside Philly
he turned and said, *My daughter has only days to live.*

Rawboned man. Under his eyes were purple crescents
like bruises dug out by a surgeon's thumb.

He wept, I was scared, but not for myself.
Of course, for myself.

I took his hand then—cold as inside of a limestone chapel.
Wilmington next. He pressed both my hands before he left.

I wanted him please
to bless me again, bless the train and the tracks for they could
    snap like

fingers like the string of smoky pearls my sweetheart gave to me
before he got sick.

Before they admitted him.
One day, on my way to the hospital, I saw some movers drop a baby
    grand—

it broke from its harness to the street.
One honors the chord of a crashed piano by scrounging ivory

for a charm.
There is logic in this.

When I walked into my sweetheart's room,
I saw the chemo had gotten to his scalp, he was ripping out

handfuls of his own hair, black dandelion seedfluff, shouting,
Take it. It doesn't even hurt.

I wound his hair round the shard of ivory to conjure the elephant
to save him. But on the train, I didn't tell the priest I had a charm

and after he left, a teenaged boy
with a ripped leather jacket took the same seat, still warm.

He looked at me staunchly: *You all right?*
I said, *My boyfriend's dead.*

Kid gave me a cigarette.
I showed the charm to him and he said

I should give it to my Mom to keep my Dad off her.
Crossing the Susquehanna, he fell asleep, twitching in a dream.

High arched brows. Eyes chasing, or being chased.
I unwound from the charm the black hair of my boyfriend,

and wrapped my own hair around it, to slip in the kid's pocket.
There was a pistol in it.

The train cut close by suburban yards
where cars roosted up on blocks, an upside-down dory perched like
    a hen

warming herself in the sun-shot dirt, a kid climbing into a tulip poplar
tore off whole blossoms to toss to his mother

as dusty babies swarmed on the grass below.
They never looked up.

All I wanted was to hear them, please
calling each other.

ELEVENTH DAY OF RAIN

Today I might see you in the hall
at work.

I could sit by you on the bench
an inch closer than Americans are
supposed to.

Your hand stretched over your book could be playing
slide guitar. Shortstop.

Fingers long as cats.

I could stop holding my breath.

How you smell is the place your neck gives onto your shoulder
where I would like to rest.

This is the eleventh day of rain in a row
when the wind off the river pimp-slaps us university whores
heading to class.

This might be the very day I see you
because I've neglected to wash my hair
and my eyes are dull as texts.

There might be five minutes.

We don't have to think
anything.

PICK IT UP

The armadillo burrows and prowls at night.
In this baby picture of this guy I like

he's frowsy with pain. Child needs to be rocked.
Armadillo resembles possum geared up to be sent to the front.

The world is wrong. If a baby cries
pick it up.

My grandmother tried to hang herself. My ma
cut her down. When this guy kisses me it's hard to catch up—

he's restless, like the kiss isn't interesting enough.
Do you think he'll forgive me if I stop?

Once I called this guy late when I had a bad dream.
He sang low on the phone a song he wrote.

Nana said she woke up in a cold locked room and didn't know
why she was alone. And this guy that I like was late for a date,

said he couldn't call 'cause who'd broken the pay phones?
Spics.

Who the hell wants to listen to that?
In my ear my mother's mouth is still saying *Slut.*

Armadillo chisels and swallows between the breasts,
feeds on bone, catches the throat and comes now

out on the step
come to repent

but if I don't stop he'll strip me, if I don't stop
he'll gloat my fat, if I don't stop, snout me in half.

He has a picture of the Buddha that for him is just an object of art.
I read that all celestial bodies turn around a central axis.

This gives me hope but I couldn't tell you why.
How can he turn and use words like that?

I had a dream my father shoved his fist inside
it woke me up. Some people so poor they must eat the armadillo

but if I had a choice, better not kill a thing.
Better not.

OLD BLOOD

In the message-carrying air…his subtlest thinking overheard…
—Herman Melville

1.

Finally April so wild struck
first night of the year with the windows up
so held and hushed in the lap of him
I became those tiny leaves
fresh as an eighth-month baby
before its shoulders are delivered
face up in the extravagant air

but then his voice got so supple and swag it slid out his kat-mouth

He wanted out

I won't say what he called me
You might crave that kind of too-sweetness
the voice gloating behind itself

I looked to his eyes to see who he suddenly was
I was fixing to beg *Don't go*

Then a song on the radio—its opening chords
walking its blues dog into me good

> *Face resist the face*
> *kind eyes where treachery's most vividly detected*
> *and your thumb you smashed in the car before you met—*
> *that nail bears a blood blister—*
> *you study that—*

The old blood was an island
                                                map in a rose ocean

2.

My cousin and I both talk too much,
to booksellers, gas station guys,
out of loneliness and worse than that

My cousin said,
the first moment you know what you'd rather not
is no time to get strange

And I said,
Spinoza thought intuition was the highest form of cognition
but he didn't say that this faculty relates to how
music can slice at a peculiar angle
so you tumble out changed in yourself,
canny as a housecat which shuns an eminent guest
because therein is a foul thing it can sense

My cousin said, Wait for me on the porch

3.

Crickets are not original
never having unlearned the one-note chant
which was your name
before you were named

so you remember what is not remembered
being an infant in arms
safe like that

which is what you wanted to be with that guy in the first place

Let the crickets knit their pulse
into your brain-silk

Follow that

FOR MY THIRD COUSIN RAY JOHN

I poured salt on slugs when I was a kid.
Foaming, they died while I watched with the thuggish
delight of a child—slight savage.
It was Ray John taught me. Two, we two
in our garbled kinhood, awash, 1956.
A small town is a boat that the wind makes a toy,
boat in a foam sea, oh the tinderbox terror of it.
Daddy's killing Mama again. What is
the impulse to save? You slugs, your killer confesses
to murder quite plain. Why was it fun?

I had to hide Ray John. The secret was
we were in the long grass. The secret now is
Ray John will die of AIDS, and soon. This
I've never told because he hurts. Me, I refuse
to bear the cross in the eyes of the nurse
who spits in the sink when I'm not looking. Looking
is something I do not enjoy. Look, any soul will do—
take mine. Because Ray John
is a better item than me or his parents.
They should be the dead ones—

                    take me,
                    not him.

I shouldn't have let him go down in that culvert when we were kids—
lie, dash, get a kiss. Away from Mama. I would save him.
Who knows where the virus diddles.
I would draw the poison as salt pulls fluid
where the wild grass grows up to cover us.
Ray John, without the dogs they'll never find us.

Lie down and pretend you're the grass of the field, Ray John,
don't cry 'cause the devil can't catch us

> *Where the workers of iniquity flourish*
> *they shall be cut down*
> *and the righteous shall grow as the cedar of Lebanon*

because I'll come back to you, never worry.
I will come right to you—
when have I not been with you—
I will lie down with you and cover you
and I will carry you into the dark dark finish.

ENDING GREEN

He thought he was smarter because he was a doctor
and I was a nurse. *Fiancé*—

the word's brainlessly soft, muckle in the mouth.
So I left him, my most excellent catch.
Left my job on the graveyard shift,
burn unit, pediatric,
kids with palms seared down to the bone
to make them stop sucking their thumbs.

Left pseudomonas—
it infects a burn,
turns it blue-green, smells morbidly sweet
and deludes some crevice inside your head
so you still smell it even after a shower,
two showers.

Forget those movies with the morgue drawers,
those private files each holding one stiff—
how exotic.

The morgue is a walk-in meat locker
with shelves like for food in your refrigerator,
only bigger.

The baby I washed and tagged and wrapped
and carried down in the freight elevator—standard procedure
—but the orderly wouldn't hold the morgue door open.

He was afeard.

I laid the baby in there on the topmost rack and pivoted quick
but the freezer door slammed shut with me inside
the chill peculiar air.

> I never thought I would pray like this,
> in a thick dark box,
> waiting for the door to turn bright

> *You Who Are   when have I not betrayed You*
> *I thought I was different from these dead*
> *Please   I'll be good*

but I always renege—
always renege.

You should have propped the door
was all my fiancé said after I got home—
I threw a can of beer at his head.
It was his voice—cool as clamps—it was his voice I quit.

I took the postcard of the Angel & the Pilgrim.
Metaphorical, but it's not.
A stranger returns your lost purse, paycheck still in it.
This you see, but the god you don't,
so you abandon hope.
You cop to pain 'cause it needs no proof,
it's how sentries talk, or your father before he slaps.
My fiancé had a voice like that.

Caught the night bus, crowded—
but the driver's cheerful with his bigarm self,
there's nothing he can't handle in this rolling coach

I just never thought the door would slam like that

Far you going? the driver says
Red Hill.
Right near me! North Garden! he says

Crossing over those dolorous hills, he tells
how his black grandmother cooked,
while the white one worked in the mill
and as he sings to himself
he smacks the note, then teases it,
rallies the feeling, then shaves it into whittles,
carries falsetto, tumbles low—
now ringing, now throaty, now grave.
Now he is pitiless with it. Then forgives.
Then lets it fade.

His voice got me to hope—
not for any man or thing
but for some kind of spirit life that I would not betray.

I sat up front and to the right of him,
rolling south-southeast over the Appalachians
into spring that is enormous and green
and goes on all day and all night.

YOU COULD HAVE BEEN ME

Just you walk out from that hospital air into the rasp edge of winter
when trees look fresh as a black lace hem
frayed in somebody's backseat.

Just walk out of the hospital, where grief is stripped and intricate
as winter trees.

I was fresh out of the sonogram room where they tilted a sensor
over and over a place in my breast.
You could have been me there—
a jacklighted deer
hearkening.

Ultrasound, imperceptible to anyone but bats,
will pass through liquid and bounce off solid
as sonar reveals a torpedo.
As it sees a malignant mass.

Doctors are whispering.

One looks over: *You mind us talking?*
Talk, I said. *Sing, if you feel like it.*

I walked straight out of that hospital
the moment the just-set-sun was casting a pearl shell over the city.

A man asked for change.
I told him the truth. I was out of work.

God bless you, he said, *come back tomorrow, I'll have money.*

My sonogram film now stood packed in with a thousand others.
When you rejoice, you forget the unspared ones.

You just watch that godlike blue between sunset and night,
blue laced with underlight curving around the shoulders of the earth
until it falls like a veil teased off—

and as a Chevy full of folks creaks down the way,
headlights swagging down the alley,
something shifts—inside me again is a perfectness.

No harm will come to us.
The street will not swallow us, the night not oppress us.

Something opens inside my chest—
a flower from a pellet in a glass of water, a toy
for a child so dumb with delight she's forgotten the difference
between herself and the one to be thanked
and the thanks, the very thanks.

THE ARGUMENT

Some people have a self-destructo streak, like a cat leaping from a
car on the interstate, or a woman getting pregnant by a jaybird of a
    lover—

a coarse-cried flash of thieving blue.
I'd long thought that little good lives in the human heart

then one lucky day I had an argument
with you. Oh

the racket I made.
Then I saw you were listening with

the most precise and startling tenderness.
This made me wonder about my assumptions.

    It was the lenient part of February
    soft with fog rising from the saturated earth,
    snowbanks turning to plumes of steam, skipping
    their intermediary state, the green in the earth biding her time.

But some people wouldn't know *hope* if it kissed them on the mouth.
Mother Tyrannosaurus locked them up inside the closet

and hissed into the keyhole—no wonder their hearts
jump out their chests. Like that cat

out the window on I-95 South—
you cut the wheel, pull off, wade into the off-road brush and call

while trucks shake the earth, mosquitoes come for you.
But even a frantic cat can see who abides in gentleness.

The sun, tilting down the sky.

                    The man, hearkening.

TO THEM, TO THEIR FIRST CONVERSATION

Sunlight: Her pituitary balks at the lack of it
and he's an engraver, so for them

light is not taken for granted. On this day in October
downtown, lunch hour, the sun's acting paternal.

Showing them off to each other. The man
is flushed with the debonair mutiny of blowing off

his day job, of loafing on the sidewalk, flirting with a woman
with bobcat green eyes. Between the edge of her scarf

and the scoop neck of her sweater there's a crescent of her skin,
unprotected. Their first conversation alone.

Blaring noon. People have to step around them.
A southeastern sky tips down to them its light,

half cloudy, like tea dashed with milk,
which, after a long illness, is brought—

slowly now—
                to the lips.

Notes

▲

Epigraphs—From Akhmatova's "A land not mine, still," translated by Jane Kenyon, in Jane Hirshfield's *Women in Praise of the Sacred.* From Vallejo's "A man walks by with a stick of bread" in Clayton Eshleman and Jose Rubia Barcia's translation, *The Complete Posthumous Poetry.*

"Baltazar Beats His Tutor at Scrabble"—Line 14 from Skakespeare's *King John.*

"An Engine Fire over the Ocean Compared to the Suburbs"—for Chuck and Dianne Hanzlicek.

"Bipolar Affective Disorder as Possible Adaptive Advantage" —Lines 28–29 from a letter by Robert Lowell to Caroline Blackwood, cited in *Creative Brainstorms: The Relationship between Madness and Genius* by Russell R. Monroe, M.D. Last six lines after Laura Jensen's "As the Window Darkens" in *Bad Boats.*

"From the Diary of a Prisoner's Nurse, Mississippi, 1972" —for Brother Mike.

"On First Hearing T'ao Ch'ien"—"The world is / boundless, boundless" from David Hinton's translation of T'ao Ch'ien, a third-century Chinese poet and forerunner of the Ch'an (Zen) poets.

"Fever, Mood, and Crows"—*Nemo censetur ignorare legem* ("No one is presumed ignorant of the law [ignorance of the law is no excuse]") cited in *The Tongue Snatchers (Les voleuses de langue)* by Claudine Herrmann, translated by Nancy Kline.

"Hear Me, Oh My Grandmothers"—Lines 39–40 from Psalm 35:10.

"Shots"—Thanks to Blas Manuel de Luna.

"Parts"—Tet: Vietnamese New Year; here, the massive North Vietnamese offensive in 1968.

"Old Blood"—Epigraph from *Moby Dick.* Last three lines after Paul Celan's "What Sews" in *Last Poems,* translated by Katharine Washburn and Margret Guillemin. Blues dog in memory of Stevie Ray Vaughan.

"For My Third Cousin Ray John"—Lines 31–33 from Psalm 92:7 and 12. Thanks to Ryan Dreimiller for the citation.

"The Argument"—for C. S.

The Author

▲

Belle Waring's first collection, *Refuge*
(University of Pittsburgh Press, 1990), won
the Associated Writing Programs' Award for
Poetry in 1989, the Washington Prize in 1991,
and was cited by *Publishers Weekly* as one of
the best books of 1990. She has received
fellowships from the National Endowment
for the Arts, the D.C. Commission on the
Arts, Virginia Center for the Creative Arts,
and the Fine Arts Work Center in
Provincetown, Massachusetts. Waring teaches
creative writing at Children's Hospital in Washington, D.C. *Dark
Blonde* has received the first annual Levis Reading Prize and the
1997 Poetry Center Book Award.

Paul Sewell